Revive Your Manhood Naturally

A Guide to Fixing Erectile Dysfunction Naturally and Safely

By Promise L. Elijah

Table Of Content

Preface
- Introduction to the Book

Chapter 1: Understanding Erectile Dysfunction
- Definition and Explanation of Erectile Dysfunction
- Prevalence and Statistics
- Causes of Erectile Dysfunction
- The Importance of Seeking Treatment

Chapter 2: Natural Approaches to Reviving Manhood
- Holistic Approach to Erectile Health
- Benefits of Natural Solutions
- Balancing Mind and Body for Improved Performance

Chapter 3: Lifestyle Changes for Erectile Health
- Diet and Nutrition
  - Essential Nutrients for Erectile Health
  - Foods to Include and Avoid
- Exercise and Physical Activity
  - Importance of Regular Exercise
  - Specific Exercises for Erectile Health
- Quality Sleep and Stress Management

- Impact of Sleep and Stress on Erectile Function
- Techniques for Stress Reduction

Chapter 4: Herbal Remedies and Supplements
- Traditional Herbs for Erectile Dysfunction
- Understanding Herbal Supplements
- Safety and Proper Usage of Herbal Remedies

Chapter 5: Natural Sexual Enhancement Techniques
- Importance of Communication with Partner
- Techniques for Intimacy and Connection
- Tips for Spicing Up Your Relationship

Chapter 6: Mindfulness and Mental Well-being
- Mind-Body Connection in Erectile Function
- Practicing Mindfulness for Enhanced Sexual Experience
- Addressing Performance Anxiety

Chapter 7: Alternative Therapies and Practices
- Acupuncture and Acupressure
- Yoga and Tai Chi for Erectile Health
- Other Complementary Practices

Chapter 8: The Role of Hormones

- Understanding Testosterone and Erectile Function
- Natural Ways to Boost Testosterone Levels
- When to Consider Hormone Therapy

Chapter 9: Creating Your Personalized Plan
- Assessing Your Current Lifestyle and Habits
- Building a Holistic Plan Tailored to Your Needs
- Tracking Progress and Making Adjustments

Conclusion

Appendix
- Additional Resources and References
- Glossary of Terms

Preface

Introduction to the Book

"Revive Your Manhood Naturally: A Guide to Fixing Erectile Dysfunction Naturally and Safely." In a world filled with quick fixes and pharmaceutical solutions, this book aims to provide a comprehensive resource for men seeking to address erectile dysfunction in a holistic and sustainable manner. Erectile dysfunction is a topic often shrouded in embarrassment and misinformation. It's a challenge that many men face, yet few openly discuss. This book seeks to change that by offering a candid and informed exploration of the subject. In the following pages, you will find a wealth of knowledge compiled from medical research, expert interviews, personal stories of triumph, and centuries-old natural remedies. Our goal is to empower you with the understanding that you have the potential to take control of your sexual health using natural approaches. We'll delve into the intricacies of erectile dysfunction, exploring both its physical and psychological origins. We'll demystify the complex relationship between lifestyle factors, hormonal balance, and sexual performance. From dietary choices to exercise routines, mindfulness practices to herbal remedies, this book covers a broad spectrum of methods that can contribute to the revival of your manhood.

By taking a proactive stance and embracing the concepts presented here, you'll embark on a journey of transformation. This is not just a guide to regaining your sexual vitality; it's an invitation to enhance your overall well-being. It's about embracing a new way of living that encompasses both physical and mental health, leading to a more fulfilling and satisfying life.

We encourage you to approach this book with an open mind and a commitment to change. Remember that you are not alone on this journey. Countless men have faced similar challenges and emerged stronger, healthier, and more confident. Their stories, along with expert insights, will serve as guiding lights as you explore the path toward revitalizing your manhood naturally and safely. As you turn the pages, absorb the knowledge within, and consider the possibilities that lie ahead. May this book serve as a trusted companion on your quest for improved erectile health and an enhanced quality of life.

Wishing you success and fulfillment on this transformative journey,

[Promise L. Elijah]

Author, "Revive Your Manhood Naturally: A Guide to Fixing Erectile Dysfunction Naturally and Safely"

1: Understanding ... Dysfunction

... dysfunction (ED) is a condition that affects ...ions of men worldwide, yet it remains widely misunderstood and often goes undiscussed. In this chapter, we will delve into the comprehensive landscape of ED, addressing its definition, prevalence, causes, and the crucial importance of seeking treatment. By gaining a thorough understanding of this condition, you will be better equipped to embark on the journey towards reviving your manhood naturally and safely.

Definition and Explanation of Erectile Dysfunction

Erectile Dysfunction (ED), often referred to as impotence, is a condition that can cast a shadow over a man's confidence and intimate relationships.

At its core, ED is characterized by the consistent inability to achieve or sustain an erection that's firm enough for sexual activity. This condition goes beyond the occasional challenges that most men face; it becomes a persistent concern that can significantly impact one's quality of life. Imagine a complex symphony of physiological and psychological factors that need to harmonize perfectly to create the beautiful melody of an erection.

ED arises when this symphony encounters discordant notes, leading to frustration and disappointment. It's a condition that transcends the physical aspect; the emotional toll can be equally profound.

Picture a scenario where a man is eager to engage in intimacy, but his body seems to betray him. The desire is present, but the response is lacking. This disparity between intention and ability can lead to feelings of inadequacy and even shame. It's essential to recognize that ED is not a reflection of one's worth or masculinity; it's a medical condition that deserves understanding and proper attention.

Understanding the mechanics of an erection provides insight into the complexity of ED. When sexual stimulation occurs, the brain sends signals that trigger a rush of blood to the penis, causing it to become erect. For men with ED, this process is hindered, either due to insufficient blood flow, nerve damage, or other physiological factors.

Moreover, the psychological element of ED cannot be ignored. Stress, anxiety, and even past negative experiences can create a cycle of apprehension that further exacerbates the condition. The mind and body are inextricably linked; disruptions in one can affect the other.

To address ED effectively, it's vital to break the cycle of silence and stigma surrounding the condition. By seeking professional guidance and exploring natural remedies, men can regain their sense of agency and rediscover the pleasure and intimacy that can flourish within relationships. Remember, the journey towards overcoming ED is not just about restoring physical function; it's about reclaiming a sense of confidence, emotional well-being, and connection.

In the pages that follow, we will delve deeper into the various facets of ED, exploring its causes, the role of lifestyle choices, and the power of natural solutions. Armed with this knowledge, you'll be equipped to navigate this intricate landscape, ultimately restoring not only your sexual vitality but also your overall sense of self-assurance.

<u>Prevalence and Statistics</u>

Understanding the prevalence of Erectile Dysfunction (ED) offers a glimpse into the far-reaching impact of this condition on men's lives. ED is not an isolated struggle; it's a widespread challenge that transcends age and cultural boundaries. Research reveals that the prevalence of ED increases with age, echoing the inevitable changes that occur within the body over time. Among men aged 40, approximately 5% experience ED. As age advances, so does the prevalence, with around 15% of men in their 50s reporting symptoms. By the age of 70, this number escalates to a staggering 50%.

These statistics underline the importance of addressing ED as a crucial aspect of men's health, particularly as longevity increases and sexual well-being remains integral to a fulfilling life.

However, it's imperative to recognize that ED is not solely an issue of aging. Younger men are not immune to its effects. A variety of factors, ranging from stress and performance anxiety to lifestyle choices and underlying health conditions, can contribute to ED at any age. These insights emphasize the need to shift the conversation around ED from one that's solely focused on older populations to one that acknowledges its presence among men of all ages.

As we navigate the path toward understanding and addressing ED, these statistics serve as a reminder that no man should feel isolated in his struggle. By acknowledging the prevalence of the condition, we foster an environment of openness and understanding, ultimately contributing to a healthier and more informed approach to managing ED. In the forthcoming chapters, we will explore the multifaceted nature of the condition, delve into its causes, and equip you with the knowledge needed to embrace a holistic strategy for revival.

Causes of Erectile Dysfunction

The intricate web of factors contributing to Erectile Dysfunction (ED) is a testament to the complexity of the human body and mind. ED is not a single-dimensional issue; it's a convergence of physical, psychological, and lifestyle elements that can impact a man's sexual vitality.

Physical Factors: Chronic medical conditions cast a significant shadow over sexual health. Conditions such as diabetes, hypertension, cardiovascular diseases, and obesity can damage blood vessels and impede the flow of blood to the penis. This disrupted blood flow hinders the process of achieving and sustaining an erection. Hormonal imbalances, particularly low testosterone levels, can also play a pivotal role in ED.

Psychological Factors: The mind's influence on sexual function is profound. Stress and anxiety can trigger a cascade of physiological responses, including the release of stress hormones that constrict blood vessels and hinder the erection process. Performance anxiety, stemming from fear of underperformance or past negative experiences, creates a self-perpetuating cycle of apprehension that can exacerbate ED.

Lifestyle Factors: Unhealthy lifestyle choices are often silent accomplices in the development of ED. Smoking, for instance, damages blood vessels, limiting the blood flow essential for achieving an erection. Excessive alcohol consumption not only impairs sexual response but also depresses the central nervous system, affecting libido. Sedentary routines and poor dietary habits contribute to obesity and cardiovascular problems, further intensifying the risk of ED.

It's essential to recognize that these factors don't exist in isolation; they often intertwine and reinforce each other. A man struggling with obesity might also battle with low self-esteem, leading to anxiety and exacerbating his ED. Similarly, a man dealing with hypertension might face stressors that further compound his condition. Understanding these interconnections underscores the importance of a holistic approach to managing ED.

Addressing the causes of ED is not just about rectifying physical symptoms; it's about embracing a comprehensive lifestyle transformation. By adopting healthy eating habits, engaging in regular exercise, and cultivating stress-reduction techniques, individuals can restore balance to their physical and mental well-being. The journey toward reviving one's manhood requires acknowledging and confronting these underlying factors, empowering men to take proactive steps in reclaiming their sexual vitality.

The Importance of Seeking Treatment

In a world where conversations about personal health can be uncomfortable, it's essential to shed light on the profound significance of seeking treatment for Erectile Dysfunction (ED). The decision to address ED is not just about enhancing sexual performance; it's a pivotal step toward improved overall well-being and relationships.

Restoring Confidence: ED can silently erode a man's self-confidence. The inability to achieve or maintain an erection can lead to feelings of inadequacy and self-doubt. Seeking treatment, whether through medical professionals or natural approaches, provides a pathway to restoring that confidence. It's about reaffirming that one's worth extends beyond their sexual function.

Strengthening Relationships: Intimacy is a cornerstone of healthy relationships. When ED enters the equation, it can strain connections between partners. The frustration and emotional distance that may result from untreated ED can ripple into other aspects of the relationship. Seeking treatment demonstrates a commitment to nurturing these connections and rekindling the emotional and physical bond between partners.

Enhancing Quality of Life: A fulfilling life encompasses physical, emotional, and mental well-being. ED can impact all these dimensions. It's not just a matter of experiencing difficulty in the bedroom; it's about the potential for a diminished quality of life. By seeking treatment, individuals can regain control over their bodies, experience improved self-esteem, and rekindle a zest for life that goes beyond the bedroom.

Addressing Underlying Issues: ED can be a symptom of underlying health conditions. Ignoring ED might mean ignoring warning signs that something more significant is at play. By seeking treatment, individuals can uncover potential health concerns and address them before they escalate into more serious problems.

Empowerment through Education: The decision to seek treatment is an empowering one. It's a declaration that one is taking charge of their health and actively seeking solutions. Knowledge is a powerful tool, and by learning about treatment options, individuals can make informed decisions that align with their values and goals.

Remember, seeking treatment for ED is not an admission of weakness; it's a statement of strength. It's a recognition that one's sexual health is an integral part of overall well-being. Whether opting for medical intervention or exploring natural remedies, the journey toward addressing ED is a journey toward self-improvement, self-acceptance, and the restoration of vitality in all facets of life. Your choice to seek treatment signifies a commitment to a healthier and more fulfilling future.

Understanding Erectile Dysfunction is the first step towards its resolution. This chapter illuminated the intricacies of ED, from its definition to prevalence, diverse causes, and the significance of seeking treatment. By comprehending the multifaceted nature of this condition, you're poised to embark on a journey of transformation. The path ahead involves addressing physical, psychological, and lifestyle factors, culminating in a holistic approach that paves the way for revived manhood and improved well-being.

Chapter 2: Natural Approaches to Reviving Manhood

In a world often dominated by pharmaceutical solutions, Chapter 2 offers a refreshing perspective on restoring erectile health naturally. This chapter delves into the holistic approach to addressing Erectile Dysfunction (ED), focusing on the benefits and principles of incorporating natural remedies into your journey towards revitalization.

Holistic Approach to Erectile Health

When it comes to addressing Erectile Dysfunction (ED), viewing it through a holistic lens opens doors to a more comprehensive and lasting solution. Holistic health acknowledges that the body is a complex system where various elements are interconnected. ED is not just a localized problem; it's a symptom that can stem from a range of factors. By embracing a holistic approach, you're not only addressing the symptom but also enhancing your overall well-being.

Physical Health: A holistic perspective recognizes the importance of physical well-being in the realm of erectile health. Engaging in regular physical activity promotes healthy blood circulation, which is essential for achieving and maintaining an erection. Moreover, maintaining a balanced diet rich in essential nutrients nourishes your body and supports optimal vascular function. A holistic approach encourages you to consider the impact of your daily choices on your sexual health.

Emotional Well-being: Stress and anxiety can create a barrier to optimal sexual function. Holistic health emphasizes the connection between emotional well-being and sexual vitality. Techniques such as mindfulness and relaxation exercises can alleviate stress, enhance self-awareness, and create a conducive mental state for intimacy. By addressing emotional factors, you're paving the way for a healthier mindset that positively influences your sexual experiences.

Relationship Dynamics: Intimacy is not solely a physical act; it's a complex interplay of emotions, trust, and communication. A holistic approach encourages open dialogues with your partner about ED, fostering a supportive environment where both individuals can collaborate on solutions. Strengthening the emotional connection can lead to more satisfying sexual experiences, transcending physical limitations.

Lifestyle Choices: Lifestyle factors encompass your daily habits, from sleep patterns to substance use. A holistic viewpoint prompts an examination of these habits and their potential impact on your sexual health. Smoking, excessive alcohol consumption, and poor sleep quality can all contribute to ED. A holistic approach encourages you to make conscious choices that align with your goals of revitalizing your sexual well-being.

Incorporating these various aspects into your approach to ED creates a comprehensive strategy that goes beyond simply addressing the symptom. By recognizing that your body and mind are intricately connected, you're empowering yourself to not only overcome ED but also enhance your overall quality of life. As you proceed through this book, remember that the holistic approach to erectile health is not just about fixing a problem; it's about embracing a lifestyle that supports your well-being on multiple levels.

Benefits of Natural Solutions

When it comes to addressing Erectile Dysfunction (ED), exploring natural solutions offers a host of benefits that extend beyond mere symptom management. Natural remedies tap into the body's inherent ability to heal and regulate, promoting lasting changes that enhance your sexual health and overall well-being.

Fewer Side Effects: One of the primary advantages of natural solutions is their tendency to have fewer side effects compared to pharmaceutical options. Natural remedies often leverage ingredients derived from plants, herbs, and minerals that have been used for centuries. This reliance on nature's offerings reduces the likelihood of adverse reactions, providing a gentler approach to achieving desired results.

Sustainable Change: Natural solutions focus on addressing underlying causes of ED rather than offering temporary relief. By targeting the root issues, such as poor blood circulation, hormonal imbalances, or psychological factors, these remedies facilitate sustainable change. This means that as you engage with natural solutions, you're not just alleviating symptoms; you're creating a foundation for improved sexual health in the long term.

Whole-Body Wellness: Natural solutions align with the concept of holistic health, which emphasizes the interconnectedness of different aspects of well-being. Many natural remedies not only target ED but also contribute to your overall health. For instance, herbs like ginseng and ginkgo biloba have been shown to enhance blood circulation, benefiting your cardiovascular system as a whole.

Empowerment and Self-Care: Embracing natural solutions empowers you to take an active role in your health. By understanding the remedies you're using, you're participating in your own well-being journey. This empowerment cultivates a sense of self-care and responsibility, contributing to an enhanced sense of control over your sexual health.

Nurturing Well-being: Natural solutions often encourage lifestyle changes that nurture overall well-being. For instance, engaging in stress-reduction techniques like meditation not only positively impacts your sexual function but also enhances your mental state and emotional resilience. This multi-faceted approach creates a ripple effect of positivity in various areas of your life. Incorporating natural solutions into your journey toward reviving your manhood is not just about addressing ED; it's about embracing a philosophy of wellness that honors your body's innate wisdom. As you explore these remedies, you're engaging in an approach that promotes sustainable change, fewer side effects, and a holistic sense of well-being. The chapters ahead will delve into specific natural remedies and techniques that empower you to harness the benefits of nature for your sexual health.

Balancing Mind and Body for Improved Performance

Achieving optimal erectile health involves more than just physical factors; it requires a harmonious balance between your mind and body. The interplay between mental and physical well-being is a crucial aspect of addressing Erectile Dysfunction (ED) naturally. By understanding and nurturing this connection, you can enhance your overall sexual performance and satisfaction.

Mindfulness and Stress Reduction: Stress can manifest physically, affecting blood flow and contributing to ED. Mindfulness techniques offer a powerful tool for managing stress and promoting relaxation. By practicing mindfulness, you're training your mind to focus on the present moment, alleviating worries about the past or future. Deep breathing exercises, meditation, and progressive muscle relaxation can all help reduce stress, fostering an environment conducive to improved sexual function.

Positive Self-Image: The way you perceive yourself plays a significant role in sexual performance. Negative self-perception, often fueled by ED, can create a self-fulfilling prophecy of underperformance. Cultivating a positive self-image involves acknowledging your strengths, focusing on what you enjoy about your body, and recognizing that ED is a medical condition, not a reflection of your worth. This mental shift can positively impact your confidence and sexual experiences.

Communication and Connection: Emotional intimacy is intimately linked to physical intimacy. Open communication with your partner about ED can alleviate the emotional burden and foster a supportive environment. By sharing your concerns, you're creating a space for understanding and collaboration. Emotional connection can enhance trust and intimacy, contributing to improved sexual satisfaction.

Visualization and Positive Imagery: The mind has a remarkable influence on the body. Visualization techniques involve creating mental images of successful and pleasurable sexual experiences. By envisioning positive outcomes, you're priming your mind and body for success. Positive imagery can alleviate performance anxiety and contribute to a more relaxed state during intimate moments.

Stress Management: Chronic stress can have a detrimental impact on sexual function. Engaging in stress-reduction practices such as regular exercise, yoga, and spending time in nature can enhance your ability to manage stress. These activities promote the release of endorphins, which are natural mood enhancers that contribute to a balanced mental state. Balancing your mind and body is not just about addressing ED; it's about embracing a lifestyle that enhances your overall well-being. By incorporating mindfulness, fostering a positive self-image, nurturing emotional connection, and managing stress, you're creating an environment that supports improved sexual performance. As you continue on your journey towards revitalizing your manhood, remember that your mind and body are powerful allies in achieving optimal sexual health. Now you know the transformative power of a holistic approach to Erectile Dysfunction. By recognizing the interconnectedness of physical health, emotional well-being, and lifestyle choices, you're equipped to embark on a journey of revival from a place of comprehensive understanding. Exploring the benefits of natural solutions unveils a path to sustainable change, reduced side effects, and enhanced overall wellness.

Moreover, mastering the art of balancing mind and body offers practical tools to manage stress, nurture self-confidence, and foster emotional connections. As you progress through the chapters ahead, remember that your commitment to a holistic approach paves the way for a revitalized manhood, improved sexual performance, and a richer quality of life. The journey you're undertaking encompasses not only the restoration of sexual vitality but also the cultivation of a harmonious and empowered existence.

Chapter 3: Lifestyle Changes for Erectile Health

Let's delves into the transformative impact of lifestyle choices on Erectile Dysfunction (ED). Recognizing that ED is often influenced by daily habits, this chapter explores how diet, exercise, sleep, and stress management can play pivotal roles in restoring and enhancing erectile health.

Diet and Nutrition

The saying "you are what you eat" holds a profound truth, especially when it comes to addressing Erectile Dysfunction (ED). Your diet plays a crucial role in supporting overall health, and this section explores how specific dietary choices can directly impact your ability to achieve and maintain a satisfying erection.

Importance of a Balanced Diet: A balanced diet is the foundation of good health, and its influence extends to your sexual vitality. The foods you consume provide essential nutrients that affect blood circulation, hormone production, and nervous system function. By nourishing your body with the right nutrients, you're promoting an environment conducive to optimal sexual performance.

Heart-Healthy Choices: Cardiovascular health is intimately linked to erectile function. The same arteries that supply blood to your heart also play a role in delivering blood to the penis. Foods that support heart health, such as fruits, vegetables, whole grains, and lean proteins, promote healthy blood vessels and enhance blood flow. By including these foods in your diet, you're improving the circulation necessary for achieving and sustaining an erection.

Limiting Processed Foods and Sugars: Processed foods and excessive sugars can contribute to obesity, diabetes, and other health conditions that increase the risk of ED. High sugar intake can lead to insulin resistance, affecting blood vessel function and hormone regulation. By moderating your consumption of processed foods and sugars, you're protecting your vascular health and reducing the risk factors associated with ED.

Omega-3 Fatty Acids: Omega-3 fatty acids, found in fatty fish, flaxseeds, and walnuts, have anti-inflammatory properties that benefit cardiovascular health. Inflammation can damage blood vessels and impair blood flow, which are critical factors in erectile function. Including omega-3-rich foods in your diet supports vascular health and contributes to improved sexual well-being.

Hydration: Adequate hydration is often overlooked but essential for overall health, including sexual health. Dehydration can affect blood viscosity, making it harder for blood to flow freely. Staying well-hydrated supports optimal blood circulation, enhancing the ability to achieve and maintain an erection.

As you embark on the journey to address ED, consider your diet as a powerful ally in your quest for improved sexual health. By embracing a balanced diet rich in heart-healthy foods, minimizing processed foods and sugars, incorporating omega-3 fatty acids, and staying hydrated, you're nurturing an environment that supports your overall well-being. The subsequent chapters will delve deeper into other lifestyle changes, exercise routines, and stress-reduction techniques that further empower you on your path to revitalized manhood.

Essential Nutrients for Erectile Health

Your body's vitality is fueled by the nutrients you provide it, and when it comes to Erectile Dysfunction (ED), specific nutrients play a pivotal role in supporting optimal sexual health. This section explores the essential nutrients that contribute to improved blood flow, hormone balance, and overall sexual function.

L-Arginine: L-Arginine is an amino acid that serves as a precursor to nitric oxide, a molecule that relaxes blood vessels and improves blood flow. This improved circulation is essential for achieving and maintaining an erection. Foods rich in L-Arginine include nuts, seeds, lean meats, and legumes. Incorporating these foods into your diet can enhance your body's production of nitric oxide, promoting healthy blood vessel function.

Zinc: Zinc is a mineral that's crucial for testosterone production and overall sexual health. Adequate levels of testosterone are essential for libido, arousal, and erectile function. Foods rich in zinc include oysters, lean meats, whole grains, and legumes. Ensuring you have sufficient zinc in your diet supports hormone balance and enhances sexual well-being.

Vitamin D: Vitamin D plays a role in various bodily functions, including maintaining healthy blood vessels. Low levels of vitamin D are linked to cardiovascular issues, which can impact blood flow to the penis. Natural sources of vitamin D include fatty fish, fortified dairy products, and sunlight exposure. Including these sources in your diet can contribute to improved cardiovascular health and erectile function.

Folate and B Vitamins: Folate and certain B vitamins are involved in energy metabolism and nerve function. Healthy nerve function is critical for sexual arousal and response. Foods rich in these nutrients include leafy greens, whole grains, and lean meats. By providing your body with the necessary building blocks for nerve health, you're supporting optimal sexual function.

Antioxidants: Antioxidants combat oxidative stress and inflammation, which can impair blood vessel function. Vitamins C and E, as well as other antioxidants found in fruits, vegetables, and nuts, contribute to overall vascular health. By including these foods in your diet, you're protecting blood vessels from damage and promoting improved blood flow.

As you cultivate a diet rich in these essential nutrients, you're fueling your body's ability to achieve and maintain healthy sexual function. By understanding the role of nutrients in promoting blood flow, hormone balance, and nerve health, you're taking a proactive step toward revitalized manhood. The subsequent chapters will delve into other lifestyle changes, exercise routines, and stress-reduction techniques that further empower you on your journey towards improved erectile health.

Foods to Include and Avoid

Making mindful choices about the foods you include in your diet can significantly impact your Erectile Dysfunction (ED) journey. This section highlights foods to embrace and avoid, shedding light on the rationale behind these choices and their influence on your sexual health.

Foods to Include:

Leafy Greens: Leafy greens like spinach, kale, and Swiss chard are rich in nitrates, compounds that support healthy blood vessel function. By improving blood flow, nitrates contribute to enhanced erectile function.

Berries: Berries, such as strawberries, blueberries, and raspberries, are packed with antioxidants that combat oxidative stress. Oxidative stress can damage blood vessels, so including berries in your diet supports vascular health.

Nuts and Seeds: Nuts and seeds, such as almonds, walnuts, and flaxseeds, provide essential fatty acids that support cardiovascular health. These healthy fats promote improved blood circulation, benefiting erectile function.

Fatty Fish: Fatty fish like salmon, mackerel, and trout are rich in omega-3 fatty acids. Omega-3s reduce inflammation, protect blood vessels, and enhance overall cardiovascular health, contributing to optimal blood flow.

Whole Grains: Whole grains, such as oats, quinoa, and brown rice, offer fiber that supports heart health. A healthy heart ensures efficient blood circulation, which is essential for achieving and sustaining an erection.

<u>Foods to Avoid:</u>

Excess Sugar: Excessive sugar consumption can lead to obesity, diabetes, and impaired blood vessel function. High sugar levels can hinder blood flow, affecting erectile function.

Processed Foods: Processed foods often contain high levels of unhealthy fats, sodium, and additives. These components can contribute to heart issues and obesity, factors that increase the risk of ED.

Saturated and Trans Fats: Saturated fats, found in red meat and full-fat dairy products, and trans fats, present in many processed foods, can contribute to artery clogging and reduced blood flow.

High Salt Intake: Excessive salt consumption can elevate blood pressure and negatively impact blood vessel health. Elevated blood pressure can contribute to ED.

Alcohol and Caffeine: While moderate alcohol consumption might not be harmful, excessive intake can impair sexual function. High caffeine consumption can lead to dehydration, affecting blood viscosity and flow.

Understanding the impact of different foods on your sexual health empowers you to make informed choices. By including nutrient-rich foods that support cardiovascular health and avoiding those that can hinder blood flow and vessel function, you're creating a diet that nurtures your overall well-being. As you progress through this chapter, consider these food guidelines as essential tools in your pursuit of revitalized erectile health.

Exercise and Physical Activity

Engaging in regular exercise isn't just about staying fit; it's a potent strategy for enhancing your Erectile Dysfunction (ED) journey. This section uncovers the significant role that exercise and physical activity play in improving blood circulation, hormonal balance, and overall sexual function.

Boosting Blood Flow: Cardiovascular exercise, such as brisk walking, jogging, cycling, and swimming, stimulates the heart and circulatory system. This increased heart rate leads to improved blood flow throughout the body, including the genital area. Enhanced blood flow to the penis is essential for achieving and maintaining an erection.

Hormonal Balance: Exercise influences hormonal balance, including testosterone levels. Testosterone is a key hormone for libido and sexual function. Engaging in regular physical activity can help maintain healthy testosterone levels, contributing to enhanced sexual well-being.

Weight Management: Obesity is a risk factor for ED, as it can contribute to cardiovascular issues, diabetes, and hormonal imbalances. Exercise helps with weight management by burning calories and promoting a healthier body composition. Maintaining a healthy weight reduces the risk of developing conditions that can lead to ED.

Stress Reduction: Physical activity is a natural stress reliever. Regular exercise triggers the release of endorphins, which are neurotransmitters that promote feelings of happiness and relaxation. By reducing stress, exercise contributes to a more positive mental state and a conducive environment for sexual arousal.

Pelvic Floor Exercises: Strengthening the pelvic floor muscles, also known as Kegel exercises, can improve erectile function. These exercises involve contracting and relaxing the muscles responsible for controlling urination and ejaculation. Pelvic floor exercises enhance blood flow to the pelvic region, supporting erectile health.

Balance and Flexibility: Yoga and stretching routines contribute to improved flexibility, posture, and balance. These benefits can enhance physical comfort during sexual activity and contribute to greater sexual satisfaction.

Moderation and Consistency: It's important to approach exercise with moderation and consistency. Overexertion can lead to injuries that might hinder your progress. Aim for regular, moderate exercise sessions that gradually increase in intensity as your fitness improves.

Cardiovascular Health: Aerobic exercises, like running, swimming, or cycling, significantly benefit your cardiovascular system. Regular cardiovascular workouts enhance heart health, improve blood vessel function, and promote efficient blood circulation. These factors are crucial for supporting erectile function by ensuring an adequate supply of blood to the penis.

By incorporating exercise into your daily routine, you're investing in your overall well-being, including your sexual health. Whether you're engaging in cardiovascular workouts, strength training, or pelvic floor exercises, each form of exercise contributes to improved blood flow, hormonal balance, and stress reduction. As you navigate through this chapter, consider exercise as a powerful tool in your quest for revitalized manhood, and embrace the positive impact it can have on your journey toward enhanced erectile function.

Importance of Regular Exercise

Beyond the physical benefits discussed earlier, the significance of regular exercise for Erectile Dysfunction (ED) encompasses a wide range of factors that contribute to improved sexual health. This section delves into the lesser-known yet equally vital reasons why incorporating regular exercise into your lifestyle can have a transformative impact on your journey towards enhanced erectile function.

Enhanced Blood Vessel Function: Exercise doesn't just improve blood circulation; it enhances the function of the blood vessels themselves. Regular physical activity promotes the production of substances that keep blood vessels flexible and responsive. This elasticity is vital for optimal blood flow, ensuring that the blood vessels dilate and constrict efficiently for sustained erection quality.

Neurotransmitter Balance: Exercise affects neurotransmitters, chemicals in the brain that play a role in mood and arousal. Regular physical activity triggers the release of dopamine, which is associated with pleasure and motivation. This enhanced neurotransmitter balance not only boosts your mood but also contributes to improved sexual desire and responsiveness.

Nerve Regeneration: Engaging in exercise stimulates the production of growth factors that support nerve regeneration. Healthy nerve function is crucial for sexual response and pleasure. By nurturing nerve health through exercise, you're enhancing your body's capacity for heightened sexual sensations and experiences.

Immune System Support: Regular exercise contributes to a stronger immune system. A robust immune system is essential for overall health, and its function extends to sexual health as well. By bolstering your immune response, you're creating an environment where your body can focus on optimizing sexual function without being compromised by infections or inflammation.

Endocrine System Regulation: Exercise has a positive impact on the endocrine system, which is responsible for hormone production and regulation. A balanced endocrine system contributes to optimal hormone levels, including testosterone. By supporting hormonal equilibrium, regular exercise ensures that your body is primed for improved sexual well-being.

Long-Term Wellness: Regular exercise is an investment in your long-term health. By prioritizing physical activity, you're reducing the risk factors for chronic conditions that can contribute to ED, such as obesity, diabetes, and cardiovascular diseases. This proactive approach to overall well-being sets the stage for a lifetime of enhanced sexual vitality.

By acknowledging these lesser-known yet significant reasons, you're expanding your understanding of why regular exercise is a cornerstone of your journey towards revitalized erectile health. Embrace exercise not only for its immediate benefits but also for its far-reaching impact on blood vessels, neurotransmitters, nerves, immunity, hormones, and your long-term well-being. As you move through this chapter, consider these nuanced aspects of exercise as powerful motivators to sustain your commitment to regular physical activity.

Specific Exercises for Erectile Health

In your quest to enhance Erectile Dysfunction (ED) naturally, specific exercises can serve as targeted tools to support blood flow, strengthen muscles, and improve overall sexual well-being. This section introduces a variety of exercises that directly contribute to revitalizing your erectile health.

Kegel Exercises: Kegel exercises target the pelvic floor muscles, which play a crucial role in maintaining erectile function and controlling ejaculation. To perform Kegels, contract and hold the muscles you would use to stop the flow of urine. Repeat this contraction for 10 seconds, then release. Aim for three sets of 10 repetitions each day.

Aerobic Workouts: Cardiovascular exercises such as jogging, cycling, swimming, and brisk walking improve blood circulation and cardiovascular fitness. These activities enhance blood flow to the genital area, promoting optimal erectile function. Aim for at least 30 minutes of moderate-intensity aerobic activity most days of the week.

Strength Training: Strength training exercises, like lifting weights or using resistance bands, enhance muscle mass and increase testosterone levels. This form of exercise supports overall hormonal balance and contributes to improved sexual health. Aim for two to three sessions per week, targeting different muscle groups.

Yoga and Stretching: Yoga and stretching routines enhance flexibility, balance, and relaxation. Specific yoga poses, like the bridge pose and the cobra pose, can increase blood flow to the pelvic region and improve sexual function. Incorporating regular stretching and yoga sessions promotes physical comfort during intimate moments.

Plank Exercises: Plank exercises engage core muscles, which support pelvic stability and overall body strength. The increased blood flow resulting from improved core strength can positively impact erectile function. Aim for three sets of 30 to 60 seconds each day.

Pilates: Pilates focuses on core strength, flexibility, and posture. Engaging in Pilates exercises like the hundred, leg circles, and the pelvic curl can enhance pelvic floor muscles and promote healthy blood flow to the genital region.

Pelvic Tilts: Pelvic tilts involve lying on your back with bent knees and tilting your pelvis to engage your core and pelvic muscles. This exercise strengthens the muscles responsible for blood flow and erection control.

Leg Raises: Leg raises target lower abdominal muscles and improve blood circulation to the pelvic area. Lie on your back, lift your legs, and lower them without letting them touch the floor. Aim for three sets of 10 repetitions.

By incorporating these specific exercises into your routine, you're taking proactive steps towards improving blood flow, muscle strength, and overall sexual function. Each exercise contributes to enhanced erectile health, promoting a revitalized sense of manhood. As you navigate through this chapter, consider these exercises as valuable tools in your holistic approach to addressing ED and fostering improved sexual well-being.

Quality Sleep and Stress Management

The significance of quality sleep and effective stress management cannot be overstated when it comes to promoting Erectile Dysfunction (ED) recovery and sexual well-being. This section delves into the crucial role that these factors play in enhancing blood flow, hormone balance, and overall sexual function.

<u>**Quality Sleep and Erectile Health:**</u>

The Sleep-Hormone Connection: Quality sleep is a cornerstone of hormonal balance. During deep sleep, the body produces testosterone, a key hormone for sexual health. Interrupted or insufficient sleep can lead to imbalances in hormone levels, potentially impacting libido and erectile function.

Restorative Power of Sleep: Quality sleep is a cornerstone of overall well-being, and its impact extends to your sexual health. During deep sleep, your body undergoes crucial repair processes, including the release of growth hormones that support tissue repair and overall vitality. These processes are essential for maintaining healthy blood vessels and erectile function.

Hormonal Balance: Sleep plays a pivotal role in regulating hormone levels, including testosterone. Testosterone is a key player in sexual desire and function. Inadequate sleep can disrupt hormone balance, potentially leading to reduced libido and erectile issues.

Improved Blood Flow: Quality sleep contributes to enhanced blood circulation, a fundamental factor in achieving and sustaining an erection. Adequate sleep supports healthy blood vessel function, ensuring efficient blood flow to the genital area during sexual arousal.

Benefits of Good Sleep: Quality sleep not only enhances physical well-being but also positively influences mood, mental clarity, and emotional resilience. Improved mood and mental health contribute to a positive sexual outlook and better sexual experiences.

Stress Management and Erectile Health:

Impact of Chronic Stress: Chronic stress triggers a cascade of physiological responses that can negatively affect sexual function. Stress releases cortisol, a hormone that can constrict blood vessels and impair blood flow, making it challenging to achieve and maintain an erection.

Mind-Body Connection: Stress is intimately connected to psychological well-being, and psychological factors significantly influence sexual health. Anxiety and worry can create performance-related stress, further exacerbating ED. Effective stress management techniques address these psychological factors, fostering a positive mindset and reducing sexual anxiety.

Relaxation and Blood Flow: Stress management techniques such as meditation, deep breathing, and progressive muscle relaxation promote relaxation and enhance blood flow. By alleviating the physical effects of stress, you're contributing to improved sexual function.

<u>**Quality Sleep and Stress Management Strategies:**</u>

Consistent Sleep Routine: Establish a regular sleep schedule by going to bed and waking up at the same times each day. Create a comfortable sleep environment that promotes restful sleep, such as a dark, quiet, and cool bedroom.

Stress Reduction Techniques: Engage in stress-reduction practices like meditation, mindfulness, and relaxation exercises. These techniques promote a calm mental state, reduce cortisol levels, and contribute to a more positive sexual experience.

Limiting Stimulants: Reduce caffeine and alcohol intake, especially close to bedtime. These substances can interfere with sleep quality and contribute to stress.

Digital Detox: Limit screen time before bed to reduce exposure to blue light, which can disrupt sleep patterns.

Engage in calming activities, such as reading or listening to soothing music, to prepare your mind for restful sleep.

Recognizing the interconnectedness of quality sleep and effective stress management is pivotal in your journey toward improved erectile health. By prioritizing adequate sleep, engaging in stress-reduction techniques, and fostering a positive mental state, you're nurturing an environment that supports optimal blood flow, hormone balance, and psychological well-being. As you progress through this chapter, consider quality sleep and stress management as invaluable tools in your arsenal for achieving revitalized manhood and enhanced sexual function.

Impact of Sleep and Stress on Erectile Function

The intricate connection between sleep, stress, and erectile function underscores the importance of nurturing these aspects for optimal sexual health. Quality sleep and effective stress management are pivotal factors that can significantly influence your ability to achieve and sustain satisfying erections.

<u>**Sleep's Influence on Erectile Function:**</u>

Hormonal Balance: During deep sleep, the body produces hormones vital for sexual health, including testosterone. Inadequate sleep can disrupt hormonal balance, potentially impacting sexual desire and performance.

Restoration and Regeneration: Sleep is a period of cellular repair and rejuvenation. Adequate sleep supports overall cardiovascular health and enhances blood vessel function, directly impacting the ability to achieve and maintain an erection.

Sleep and Mood: Quality sleep contributes to improved mood and mental clarity. A positive mental state is essential for sexual arousal and overall sexual satisfaction.

Stress's Influence on Erectile Function:

Blood Vessel Constriction: Chronic stress triggers the release of stress hormones, leading to the constriction of blood vessels. This constriction impedes blood flow, which is crucial for a successful erection.

Mind-Body Connection: Stress management techniques foster a harmonious relationship between the mind and body. A relaxed mental state creates an environment conducive to sexual arousal and performance.

Stress and Performance Anxiety: High stress levels can exacerbate performance anxiety, creating a cycle that negatively impacts sexual function. Effective stress management breaks this cycle and promotes relaxation during intimate moments.

Recognizing the profound influence of sleep and stress on erectile function empowers you to make conscious lifestyle choices that support sexual well-being. By prioritizing quality sleep, you're promoting hormonal balance, cardiovascular health, and mood enhancement. Engaging in stress management techniques creates a mental state that promotes relaxation and reduces the physiological impact of stress on blood vessels.

As you navigate through this chapter, consider the impact of sleep and stress on your journey towards revitalized sexual health. By nurturing these aspects, you're not only addressing the physical factors that contribute to ED but also creating a holistic approach that supports your overall well-being and sexual satisfaction.

Techniques for Stress Reduction

Effectively managing stress is a cornerstone of promoting optimal Erectile Dysfunction (ED) recovery and overall sexual well-being. This section explores a range of proven techniques that can empower you to navigate stressors and foster a more relaxed and conducive mental environment for enhanced sexual function.

Biofeedback: Biofeedback involves using technology to monitor and gain awareness of physiological responses to stress, such as heart rate and muscle tension. Learning to control these responses can empower you to regulate your body's reactions to stressors, promoting relaxation and reducing the negative impact on blood vessels and sexual function.

Progressive Muscle Relaxation: This technique involves systematically tensing and then relaxing different muscle groups, promoting a sense of physical and mental relaxation. Regular practice of progressive muscle relaxation can reduce muscle tension, alleviate stress, and contribute to a more serene mental state.

Visualization: Guided imagery and visualization techniques involve creating mental images of peaceful and calming scenarios. By immersing yourself in these positive mental landscapes, you're promoting relaxation and reducing the physiological effects of stress on blood vessels.

Mindful Breathing: Mindful breathing techniques focus on deep, slow, and intentional breaths. As you direct your attention to your breath, you're cultivating mindfulness, which counters stress by redirecting your focus away from worry and anxiety.

Tai Chi and Qigong: These ancient practices combine movement, breath, and meditation to promote relaxation and balance in both the body and mind. Engaging in Tai Chi or Qigong sessions can foster physical and mental equilibrium, reducing stress and creating an optimal state for sexual well-being.

Journaling: Expressing your thoughts and feelings through journaling provides an outlet for processing stress and emotions. Journaling can help you gain insights into stressors and develop strategies for coping, fostering emotional resilience.

Guided Meditation: Guided meditation involves listening to a recorded meditation that leads you through relaxation and visualization exercises. These sessions provide guidance and structure, making meditation accessible for beginners and those looking to deepen their practice.

Each technique offers a unique approach to stress reduction, equipping you with valuable tools to combat the negative impact of stress on erectile function. By incorporating these techniques into your daily routine, you're fostering a mindset of calmness, resilience, and relaxation. As you progress through this chapter, consider these stress reduction strategies as essential elements of your holistic approach to enhancing sexual well-being and addressing ED.

Chapter 4: Natural Remedies and Supplements for Erectile Health

We take a delve into the realm of natural remedies and supplements that can play a supportive role in revitalizing your Erectile Dysfunction (ED) journey. Exploring herbal solutions, vitamins, and minerals, this chapter provides insights into how these natural interventions can enhance blood flow, hormone balance, and overall sexual function.

Traditional Herbs for Erectile Dysfunction

For centuries, various cultures have turned to traditional herbs as natural remedies to address Erectile Dysfunction (ED) and enhance sexual well-being. This section explores a range of traditional herbs that have gained recognition for their potential to improve blood flow, boost libido, and support optimal erectile function.

Panax Ginseng: Also known as Asian ginseng, Panax ginseng has a history of use as an adaptogen, helping the body adapt to stress and promote overall vitality. Research suggests that Panax ginseng may enhance nitric oxide production, leading to improved blood circulation and better erectile function.

Horny Goat Weed (Epimedium): This herb has been used in traditional Chinese medicine for its aphrodisiac properties. It contains icariin, a compound that has shown potential in increasing blood flow to the penis and enhancing erectile response.

Tribulus Terrestris: Widely used in Ayurvedic medicine, Tribulus Terrestris is believed to support hormonal balance and enhance sexual desire. Some studies suggest that this herb may boost testosterone levels, contributing to improved libido and sexual performance.

Maca Root: Native to the Andes region, Maca root has been used traditionally to enhance fertility and libido. It's rich in vitamins, minerals, and amino acids that support overall well-being, including sexual function.

Yohimbe: Derived from the bark of an African tree, Yohimbe has been traditionally used as an aphrodisiac. It contains yohimbine, a compound that can dilate blood vessels and enhance blood flow to the penis. However, caution is advised due to potential side effects.

Ashwagandha: A staple in Ayurvedic medicine, Ashwagandha is an adaptogenic herb known for its stress-reducing properties. By reducing stress, Ashwagandha indirectly supports hormone balance and may contribute to improved sexual function.

Ginkgo Biloba: Known for its ability to enhance blood circulation, Ginkgo Biloba may improve blood flow to the genital region, aiding in achieving and maintaining erections. It also has antioxidant properties that protect blood vessels from damage.

Saw Palmetto: Often used for prostate health, Saw Palmetto may also support sexual function by promoting hormonal balance. It's believed to inhibit the conversion of testosterone into dihydrotestosterone (DHT), a hormone that can contribute to ED.

Damiana: Native to Central and South America, Damiana has a long history of use as an aphrodisiac. It's believed to enhance sexual desire and performance by increasing blood flow to the pelvic region and promoting relaxation.

Muira Puama: Often referred to as "potency wood," Muira Puama is a Brazilian herb used to support sexual health. It's believed to enhance libido, improve erectile function, and alleviate symptoms of ED.

Saffron: This exotic spice has been associated with improved sexual function and enhanced mood. Research suggests that saffron may have a positive impact on serotonin levels, promoting feelings of pleasure and reducing stress.

Cnidium Monnieri: Commonly used in traditional Chinese medicine, Cnidium Monnieri is believed to promote the release of nitric oxide, a vasodilator that enhances blood flow to the genital region. This increased blood flow supports optimal erectile function.

Gokshura (Tribulus terrestris): In Ayurvedic medicine, Gokshura is used to improve sexual health and fertility. It's believed to enhance testosterone levels, leading to improved libido and better erectile function.

<u>Consultation and Caution</u>

While traditional herbs offer potential benefits, it's important to approach their use with caution. Consultation with a healthcare professional is advised, especially if you have underlying health conditions or are taking medications. Individual responses to these herbs may vary, and interactions with other medications should be considered. By exploring traditional herbs, you're tapping into nature's offerings to support your ED journey. These herbs have been valued for generations for their potential to enhance blood flow, boost libido, and contribute to optimal erectile function. As you navigate through this chapter, consider the knowledge of traditional herbs as a valuable resource in your holistic approach to addressing ED and fostering improved sexual well-being.

Understanding Herbal Supplements

As you embark on your journey to address Erectile Dysfunction (ED) naturally, understanding herbal supplements is essential to making informed and effective choices for your sexual well-being. This section provides insights into the world of herbal supplements, shedding light on their mechanisms of action, potential benefits, and considerations.

Herbal Supplements and Erectile Health:

Mechanisms of Action: Herbal supplements for ED often work by enhancing blood flow, promoting hormonal balance, reducing stress, and supporting overall sexual function. These supplements contain bioactive compounds that interact with the body to produce specific effects.

Potential Benefits: Herbal supplements offer potential benefits such as improved blood circulation to the genital region, enhanced libido, reduced stress and anxiety, and support for hormone production. Some supplements may also contribute to increased energy and stamina, promoting a more satisfying sexual experience.

Considerations for Choosing Supplements:

Research and Quality: When considering herbal supplements, prioritize those that have undergone scientific research and quality testing. Look for reputable brands that adhere to good manufacturing practices.

Dosage and Guidelines: Follow recommended dosage guidelines provided on the supplement packaging or as advised by a healthcare professional. Start with the lowest effective dose and gradually increase if necessary.

Consultation: Before incorporating herbal supplements into your regimen, consult a healthcare provider. This is especially important if you have underlying health conditions, are taking medications, or are at risk for interactions.

Potential Side Effects: Herbal supplements can cause side effects or interact with medications. Be aware of possible adverse effects and interactions, and monitor your body's response.

Understanding herbal supplements empowers you to make informed choices that align with your ED journey. By considering mechanisms of action, potential benefits, and safety guidelines, you can integrate herbal supplements into your natural approach to addressing ED and fostering improved sexual well-being. As you navigate through this chapter, view herbal supplements as valuable tools in your holistic strategy for revitalizing your sexual health.

Safety and Proper Usage of Herbal Remedies

When exploring herbal remedies as a natural approach to addressing Erectile Dysfunction (ED), prioritizing safety and proper usage is paramount. This section provides comprehensive guidance to ensure that you make informed decisions, minimize risks, and optimize the benefits of herbal remedies for your sexual well-being.

Research and Education:

Evidence-Based Information: Seek information from reputable sources such as scientific studies, clinical trials, and credible medical websites. Reliable research provides insights into the effectiveness, mechanisms, and potential risks of herbal remedies.

Consult Healthcare Professionals: Before incorporating herbal remedies into your regimen, consult a qualified healthcare provider. This is especially crucial if you have pre-existing health conditions, are taking medications, or are at risk for interactions.

Quality Assurance: Choose herbal remedies from reputable brands that adhere to good manufacturing practices. Look for supplements with standardized extracts and quality testing to ensure you're getting the intended dose and potency.

<u>**Dosage and Usage:**</u>

Follow Guidelines: Adhere to the recommended dosage and usage guidelines provided on the supplement packaging or as advised by your healthcare provider. Starting with a lower dose and gradually increasing if necessary can help minimize potential side effects.

Consistency: Consistency is key to experiencing the potential benefits of herbal remedies. Follow the recommended dosing schedule consistently to achieve optimal results.

Duration: Some herbal remedies may take time to show noticeable effects. Be patient and allow sufficient time for the compounds to build up in your system and produce results.

Potential Risks and Interactions:

Individual Variability: Responses to herbal remedies can vary based on factors such as genetics, overall health, and medication use. Monitor your body's response and be vigilant for any adverse effects.

Medication Interactions: Certain herbal remedies can interact with medications, leading to unwanted effects or reducing the efficacy of prescription drugs. Inform your healthcare provider about any herbal supplements you're considering.

Side Effects: While many herbal remedies are generally safe, some individuals may experience side effects such as digestive disturbances, allergic reactions, or changes in blood pressure. Be attentive to any changes in how you feel and consult a healthcare provider if necessary.

Long-Term Considerations:

Balanced Approach: While herbal remedies offer potential benefits, they're just one component of a holistic approach to addressing ED. Combining herbal remedies with lifestyle adjustments, stress management, and communication strategies can provide comprehensive support.

Regular Check-Ins: Periodically review your use of herbal remedies with your healthcare provider. This allows you to assess their effectiveness, make any necessary adjustments, and ensure they align with your overall health goals.

By prioritizing safety and proper usage, you're optimizing the potential benefits of herbal remedies while minimizing risks. Embrace a cautious and informed approach, consulting healthcare professionals, and staying well-educated about the herbal remedies you choose. As you navigate through this chapter, consider safety and proper usage as fundamental principles in your journey toward revitalized erectile health and enhanced sexual well-being.

Chapter 5: Natural Sexual Enhancement Techniques

Let's take a ride into the realm of natural sexual enhancement techniques that transcend physical factors, focusing on emotional intimacy, communication, and strategies to strengthen your relationship. By fostering a deeper connection with your partner and exploring techniques that promote intimacy, you're creating a holistic approach to addressing Erectile Dysfunction (ED) and enhancing your sexual well-being.

Importance of Communication with Partner

Open and honest communication with your partner is a cornerstone of nurturing a satisfying and fulfilling sexual relationship. Effective communication not only creates an environment of trust and understanding but also addresses any emotional barriers that might contribute to ED.

Creating a Safe Space: Establish a safe and non-judgmental space for discussing concerns, fears, and desires. Encourage your partner to share their thoughts as well, fostering a reciprocal exchange of feelings.

Discussing Expectations: Openly discuss each other's expectations and desires when it comes to intimacy. Understanding each other's needs helps set realistic expectations and fosters a sense of mutual respect.

Addressing Emotional Factors: Emotional factors such as stress, anxiety, and past experiences can contribute to ED. By sharing your feelings and experiences, you and your partner can work together to address any emotional barriers.

Seeking Solutions Together: Approach ED as a shared challenge rather than an individual struggle. Involve your partner in exploring potential solutions and strategies to enhance your sexual experiences.

Techniques for Intimacy and Connection

Intimacy goes beyond physical contact—it involves emotional connection, vulnerability, and shared experiences. This section explores techniques that promote emotional intimacy and strengthen your bond with your partner.

Embrace Emotional Vulnerability: Share your thoughts, fears, and desires with your partner. Being emotionally vulnerable fosters a deeper sense of connection and promotes understanding.

Sensate Focus: Sensate focus exercises involve touching and exploring each other's bodies in a non-sexual manner. These exercises promote sensual awareness and help you connect on a deeper level.

Quality Time: Spend quality time together engaging in activities you both enjoy. Whether it's a walk, cooking a meal together, or watching a movie, these shared experiences strengthen your emotional connection.

Practice Active Listening: When your partner shares their thoughts and feelings, practice active listening. This demonstrates your attentiveness and reinforces a sense of being heard and understood.

Tips for Spicing Up Your Relationship

Maintaining excitement and novelty in a long-term relationship is essential for keeping the spark alive. This section provides tips to rekindle passion and add a touch of spontaneity to your relationship.

Explore New Activities: Engaging in new activities together can infuse your relationship with fresh energy. Whether it's trying a new hobby or taking a spontaneous day trip, shared experiences create lasting memories.

Surprise Gestures: Surprise your partner with thoughtful gestures a handwritten note, a small gift, or a spontaneous date night. These gestures show your appreciation and keep the romance alive.

Flirtation and Teasing: Playful flirtation and teasing can add a sense of fun and anticipation to your interactions. Keeping things light-hearted and engaging contributes to a vibrant and exciting relationship.

Change of Scenery: Switch up your routine by planning a getaway or even a simple weekend retreat. A change of scenery can rejuvenate your connection and provide a fresh perspective.

As you immerse yourself in Chapter 5, consider these techniques as powerful tools to cultivate emotional intimacy, enhance communication, and infuse your relationship with excitement. By prioritizing emotional connection, vulnerability, and shared experiences, you're fostering an environment that supports not only improved sexual function but also a deeper, more satisfying connection with your partner.

Chapter 6: Mindfulness and Mental Well-being

Let's look at the profound impact of mindfulness and mental well-being on Erectile Dysfunction (ED) recovery and overall sexual health. By exploring the mind-body connection, practicing mindfulness, and addressing performance anxiety, you're equipping yourself with invaluable tools to foster a balanced and positive approach to sexual experiences.

Mind-Body Connection in Erectile Function

The intricate interplay between the mind and the body goes beyond physicality, extending its influence into the realm of sexual function. In this section, we explore the fascinating mind-body connection and its pivotal role in Erectile Dysfunction (ED) and overall sexual health. Understanding the psychological factors that impact erectile function empowers you to cultivate a holistic approach that addresses both the physical and mental aspects of sexual well-being.

<u>**Psychological Factors and Erectile Function:**</u>

Stress and Anxiety: The mind's response to stress and anxiety can have a profound impact on blood flow and hormonal balance. Chronic stress triggers the release of stress hormones, constricting blood vessels and reducing blood flow to the genital region. This constriction can impede the ability to achieve and maintain an erection.

Negative Emotions: Feelings of depression, low self-esteem, and negative self-perception can create a cycle that perpetuates erectile difficulties. Negative emotions can lead to a lack of interest in sexual activity, further contributing to ED.

Performance Anxiety: The fear of not meeting expectations or experiencing difficulties during sexual encounters can lead to performance anxiety. This anxiety triggers physiological responses that interfere with relaxation and optimal blood flow.

Neurological Pathways and Sexual Arousal:

The brain plays a central role in the process of sexual arousal. When the brain perceives sensory stimuli, emotions, or fantasies, it initiates a complex cascade of neurological responses that influence sexual function.

Hormonal Release: The brain's response to sexual stimuli triggers the release of hormones and neurotransmitters that play a key role in erectile function. These include dopamine, oxytocin, and nitric oxide, which impact blood flow, relaxation, and overall sexual response.

Positive Mindset and Enhanced Erectile Function:

Cultivating a positive mindset is essential for fostering a healthy sexual response. Positive emotions, self-confidence, and a strong self-image contribute to improved sexual experiences and overall sexual health.

Confidence: Confidence in your own sexual abilities and self-image can positively impact sexual function. Self-assuredness reduces performance anxiety and allows you to focus on the moment.

Positive Outlook: A positive outlook on sexual experiences can lead to increased relaxation and heightened sensations. This positive frame of mind creates an environment conducive to achieving and maintaining erections.

Emotional Connection: Emotional intimacy with your partner enhances the mind-body connection. A strong emotional bond can alleviate stress, reduce performance anxiety, and promote optimal sexual response.

Recognizing the profound influence of the mind on erectile function underscores the importance of addressing both physical and psychological factors when seeking to improve sexual well-being. By fostering a positive mindset, managing stress, and addressing emotional barriers, you're creating a holistic approach that supports not only optimal erectile function but also overall mental and emotional wellness. As you navigate through this chapter, consider the mind-body connection as a foundational element of your journey toward revitalized sexual health.

Practicing Mindfulness for Enhanced Sexual Experience

Mindfulness, the practice of being fully present in the moment, offers profound benefits for sexual well-being. By integrating mindfulness into your approach to intimacy, you're enhancing connection, reducing stress, and fostering a deeper sense of presence.

Sensual Awareness and Mindful Touch:

Mindfulness encourages you to engage all your senses during intimate moments, creating a deeper connection with your partner and your own sensations.

Focus on Touch: Pay close attention to the sensations of touch during intimate moments. Notice the textures, temperatures, and pressures as you and your partner engage in physical contact.

Slow and Deliberate Movements: Embrace slow and deliberate movements during foreplay and intimate encounters. Mindful movements allow you to savor each sensation and promote a heightened state of arousal.

Relinquishing Distractions: Mindfulness involves letting go of distracting thoughts and worries. Redirect your attention to the sensations, sights, and sounds of the present moment, immersing yourself fully in the experience.

Reducing Performance Anxiety:

Mindfulness techniques can alleviate performance anxiety by shifting your focus away from outcomes and redirecting it to the present moment.

Centering on Breath: Focus on your breath to stay grounded and present during intimate moments. Deep, steady breaths help calm the nervous system and reduce anxiety.

Being in the Moment: Redirect your thoughts from future outcomes to the sensations and emotions you're experiencing right now. Embrace the pleasure of the present moment without the weight of expectations.

Enhancing Emotional Connection:

Mindfulness promotes emotional intimacy by creating a space for open communication and mutual vulnerability.

Deepening Connection: Maintain eye contact and engage in open conversations before, during, and after sexual encounters. Sharing your thoughts and feelings fosters a deeper emotional bond.

Non-Judgmental Attitude: Approach sexual experiences without judgment or criticism. Mindfulness encourages acceptance of your own and your partner's desires, responses, and expressions.

Creating a Mindful Ritual:

Incorporate mindfulness into your daily routine to cultivate a sense of presence and anticipation for intimate moments.

Mindful Rituals: Engage in mindfulness practices outside of sexual encounters, such as meditation, deep breathing, or body scan exercises. These practices help you remain attuned to your own sensations and emotions.

Anticipating Pleasure: By embracing mindfulness throughout your day, you create a state of anticipation and excitement for the intimate moments to come.

Embracing mindfulness techniques enhances your ability to be fully present, relish sensations, and reduce performance anxiety. By immersing yourself in the present moment, you're fostering a deeper connection with your partner and creating an environment of relaxation and emotional intimacy. As you navigate through this chapter, consider mindfulness as a powerful tool to enhance your sexual experiences, cultivate emotional connection, and contribute to your journey toward revitalized sexual well-being.

Addressing Performance Anxiety

Performance anxiety is a common concern that can significantly impact sexual well-being, contributing to Erectile Dysfunction (ED) and hindering overall sexual satisfaction. This section delves into the intricate aspects of performance anxiety, offering insights, strategies, and practical approaches to overcome this barrier and enhance your sexual experiences.

Understanding Performance Anxiety:
Performance anxiety arises from the fear of not meeting expectations or experiencing difficulties during sexual encounters. This fear can trigger physiological responses that interfere with relaxation and optimal sexual function.

Psychological Impact: Anxiety and stress can lead to elevated levels of adrenaline and cortisol, which constrict blood vessels and hinder the natural flow of blood to the genital area, making it difficult to achieve and maintain an erection.

Negative Cycle: The fear of failure can create a self-perpetuating cycle. Worrying about potential difficulties increases anxiety, leading to more significant challenges during sexual experiences.

Effective Strategies for Overcoming Performance Anxiety:

Open Communication: Discuss your concerns with your partner in an open and honest manner. Sharing your feelings fosters a supportive environment that alleviates the pressure of performance.

Shift Focus: Redirect your attention away from the outcome and toward the present moment. Embrace mindfulness techniques to remain fully engaged in the sensations and emotions of the experience.

Change Perspective: Challenge negative thought patterns. Replace self-critical thoughts with affirmations that promote self-confidence and a positive outlook on sexual encounters.

Progressive Desensitization: Gradually expose yourself to sexual situations that evoke anxiety. By incrementally increasing exposure, you build resilience and decrease the intensity of anxiety responses.

Relaxation Techniques: Practice relaxation exercises, such as deep breathing and progressive muscle relaxation, to counteract the physiological effects of anxiety. These techniques promote overall relaxation and help manage stress.

Mindfulness and Sensual Focus:

Mindful Presence: Engage in sensual awareness exercises, such as sensate focus. These exercises encourage you and your partner to explore each other's bodies without the pressure of performance.

Shared Exploration: By focusing on mutual pleasure rather than individual performance, you create an environment that supports emotional connection and reduces anxiety.

Professional Support: Seek guidance from therapists, counselors, or sexologists who specialize in sexual health. Professional support offers personalized strategies and tools for managing performance anxiety.

Patience and Self-Compassion:
Overcoming performance anxiety requires patience and self-compassion. Remember that it's normal to experience occasional challenges, and setbacks are part of the journey toward enhanced sexual well-being.

Addressing performance anxiety is a crucial step toward revitalizing sexual experiences and promoting erectile health. By employing strategies such as open communication, mindfulness, relaxation techniques, and professional support, you can break the cycle of anxiety and create an environment conducive to a more satisfying and fulfilling sexual life. Embrace the journey toward overcoming performance anxiety as an opportunity to cultivate self-confidence, deepen emotional connection, and embrace a holistic approach to sexual well-being.

Chapter 7: Alternative Therapies and Practices

In Chapter 7, we delve into the world of alternative therapies and practices that offer unique avenues for addressing Erectile Dysfunction (ED) and promoting sexual well-being. From ancient healing traditions to modern complementary approaches, this chapter explores how acupuncture, acupressure, yoga, tai chi, and other practices can play a role in enhancing erectile health and overall sexual vitality.

Acupuncture and Acupressure

The ancient healing practices of acupuncture and acupressure offer intriguing possibilities for addressing Erectile Dysfunction (ED) and promoting overall well-being. Rooted in traditional Chinese medicine, these modalities are based on the belief that the body's vital energy, or "Qi," flows along specific pathways called meridians. By targeting key points along these meridians, acupuncture and acupressure aim to restore balance and encourage the body's innate healing mechanisms.

Acupuncture: Acupuncture involves the precise insertion of thin needles into specific points on the body's meridians. This stimulates the flow of Qi, facilitating improved circulation, energy balance, and relaxation. For ED, acupuncture may enhance blood flow to the genital region and address underlying imbalances that contribute to sexual health issues.

Acupressure: Acupressure shares similarities with acupuncture but uses pressure instead of needles to stimulate meridian points. By applying gentle yet firm pressure using fingers, palms, or specialized tools, acupressure aims to release tension, promote relaxation, and alleviate various ailments, including stress-related concerns that can impact sexual function.

Potential Benefits for ED:

1. Enhanced Circulation: Both acupuncture and acupressure are thought to promote blood circulation throughout the body, including to the pelvic region. Improved blood flow is crucial for achieving and maintaining erections.

2. Stress Reduction: Chronic stress and anxiety can contribute to ED. Acupuncture and acupressure's relaxation-inducing effects help reduce stress hormones, thereby fostering an environment conducive to sexual function.

3. Balancing Energy: According to traditional Chinese medicine, imbalances in Qi can lead to health issues. Acupuncture and acupressure aim to restore balance in the body's energy flow, potentially addressing the root causes of ED.

Practical Application:

Acupressure can be integrated into self-care routines for ongoing support. By familiarizing yourself with specific acupressure points associated with sexual vitality, you can apply pressure in a gentle and deliberate manner to promote relaxation and improved blood circulation.

Regular practice may help you address both physical and emotional factors that impact your sexual well-being.

<u>Consultation and Safety:</u>

If you're considering acupuncture, seeking the expertise of a licensed acupuncturist is essential. A qualified practitioner can assess your specific needs and tailor treatments accordingly. Similarly, with acupressure, understanding the correct pressure points and techniques is crucial to avoid potential discomfort or adverse effects.

As you explore the potential benefits of acupuncture and acupressure for ED, keep in mind that these practices are just one facet of a comprehensive approach to sexual health. By integrating these modalities with insights from other chapters, such as lifestyle adjustments, communication strategies, and mindfulness techniques, you're embracing a multifaceted approach that supports optimal erectile function and overall well-being.

Yoga and Tai Chi for Erectile Health

The ancient practices of yoga and tai chi offer not only physical benefits but also holistic approaches to enhancing Erectile Dysfunction (ED) and overall well-being. Rooted in mindful movement and breath control, these practices provide valuable tools for addressing both the physical and emotional aspects of sexual health.

Yoga:

Physical Movements: Yoga encompasses a range of postures and movements that promote flexibility, strength, and balance. Certain poses, such as those that engage the pelvic floor muscles and open the hips, can enhance blood flow to the genital area and contribute to improved erectile function.

Stress Reduction: Chronic stress can negatively impact sexual health. Yoga's emphasis on relaxation, deep breathing, and mindfulness can help reduce stress hormones, leading to a more relaxed and pleasurable sexual experience.

Body Awareness: Yoga encourages a heightened awareness of the body, which can foster a positive body image and improve self-confidence. This shift in self-perception can contribute to a more satisfying sexual relationship.

Tai Chi:

Gentle Movement: Tai chi is characterized by slow and flowing movements that engage the entire body. This gentle exercise promotes circulation, flexibility, and balance, supporting overall physical vitality.

Stress Reduction: Similar to yoga, tai chi's meditative aspect encourages relaxation and reduces stress. By calming the mind and nervous system, tai chi can alleviate performance anxiety and improve sexual responsiveness.

Mind-Body Connection: Tai chi emphasizes the connection between the mind and the body. Practicing tai chi enhances body awareness and fosters a greater understanding of how mental and emotional states influence physical well-being.

Integration for Erectile Health:

Integrating yoga and tai chi into your routine can contribute to enhanced sexual health and a more fulfilling intimate life.

Customization: Both practices can be tailored to your fitness level and needs. Consult with experienced instructors to create routines that address your specific concerns and goals.

Consistency: Regular practice is key to experiencing the benefits of yoga and tai chi. Consistency promotes flexibility, relaxation, and improved blood circulation over time.

Mindful Presence: Engaging in yoga and tai chi requires being fully present in the moment. This attentiveness promotes mindfulness during intimate moments, leading to a more satisfying and fulfilling sexual experience.

Holistic Approach: Incorporating yoga and tai chi into your lifestyle complements other strategies explored in earlier chapters. By fostering physical vitality, stress reduction, and emotional balance, these practices contribute to a comprehensive approach to addressing ED.

As you explore the practices of yoga and tai chi, recognize that their benefits extend beyond physical well-being. By embracing these ancient traditions, you're fostering a mind-body connection that supports enhanced erectile health and a more holistic approach to sexual vitality.

Other Complementary Practices

In addition to acupuncture, acupressure, yoga, and tai chi, a variety of other complementary practices offer unique avenues for addressing Erectile Dysfunction (ED) and promoting overall sexual well-being. These practices encompass a range of techniques that focus on relaxation, mindfulness, and overall physical vitality, contributing to a holistic approach to sexual health.

Meditation:

Stress Reduction: Meditation is a practice that cultivates mental clarity and relaxation. By quieting the mind and focusing on the present moment, meditation reduces stress and anxiety, fostering an environment conducive to sexual well-being.

Mindfulness: Mindfulness meditation enhances self-awareness and presence. By staying attuned to your sensations, emotions, and thoughts, you're better equipped to address potential barriers to sexual satisfaction.

<u>**Herbal Supplements:**</u>

Complementary Support: Certain herbal supplements, previously explored in the book, can complement other practices by promoting blood circulation, hormonal balance, and overall sexual vitality.

Quality Assurance: When considering herbal supplements, prioritize high-quality products from reputable sources. Consult healthcare professionals to ensure compatibility with your health status and any medications you're taking.

<u>**Breathing Exercises:**</u>

Deep Breathing: Specific breathing techniques, such as deep abdominal breathing, encourage relaxation and oxygenation of the body. Improved oxygen flow can positively impact blood circulation and contribute to better sexual responsiveness.

Relaxation Breathing: Techniques like relaxation breathing promote a state of calmness and reduce anxiety. Incorporating these practices into your daily routine can create an environment of ease and readiness for sexual encounters.

Holistic Integration:

While individually valuable, these complementary practices are most effective when integrated into a holistic approach to addressing ED and fostering sexual well-being.

Customization: Each practice can be tailored to your preferences and needs. Experiment with different techniques to find those that resonate most with you.

Combination: Combining practices, such as meditation and breathing exercises, can amplify their benefits. For instance, practicing deep breathing during meditation sessions enhances relaxation and supports improved sexual function.

Long-Term Benefits: Consistent engagement with these complementary practices contributes to lasting improvements in stress management, body awareness, and overall vitality—factors that are crucial for addressing ED.

Personal Exploration: As you explore these practices, remember that personal preference and individual responses play a role. What works for one person might differ for another, so be open to adapting and adjusting based on your unique needs and experiences.

By incorporating these complementary practices into your routine, you're nurturing a holistic approach to sexual well-being that encompasses physical vitality, mental clarity, and emotional balance. As you integrate these practices alongside the insights gained from earlier chapters, you're fostering a comprehensive journey toward revitalized erectile health and a more fulfilling sexual life.

Chapter 8: The Role of Hormones

Let's take a journey into the intricate role of hormones in Erectile Dysfunction (ED) and overall sexual health. Hormones, particularly testosterone, play a pivotal role in male sexual function. This chapter explores the relationship between testosterone and erectile function, outlines natural methods to boost testosterone levels, and discusses the considerations surrounding hormone therapy.

Understanding Testosterone and Erectile Function

Testosterone, often recognized as the primary male sex hormone, serves as a crucial foundation for male sexual health and function. This section offers a comprehensive exploration of the intricate relationship between testosterone and erectile function, shedding light on the pivotal role this hormone plays in maintaining optimal sexual vitality.

Hormonal Influence on Sexual Health:

Testosterone operates as a master regulator of various bodily functions, extending its influence to sexual desire, erectile quality, and overall sexual well-being.

Sexual Desire (Libido): Adequate testosterone levels are essential for maintaining a healthy libido. This hormone fosters the desire for sexual activity and ignites the spark of intimacy between partners.

Erectile Quality: Testosterone supports the mechanisms necessary for achieving and sustaining erections. It promotes the release of nitric oxide, a molecule that relaxes blood vessel walls and allows for increased blood flow to the penile region—an integral factor in erectile function.

Hormone Balance and Blood Flow: Testosterone contributes to balanced blood flow throughout the body, including the genital area. Optimal blood flow is vital for engorgement of the erectile tissues and the firmness required for satisfactory sexual encounters.

Age and Testosterone Decline:

As men age, testosterone levels tend to decrease naturally. This decline, often referred to as "andropause" or "male menopause," can impact sexual health and function.

Reduced Libido: Lower testosterone levels are associated with decreased libido, leading to changes in sexual desire and arousal.

Erectile Difficulties: A decline in testosterone can contribute to challenges in achieving and maintaining erections. This can affect not only sexual satisfaction but also self-esteem and overall well-being.

Addressing Hormonal Shifts: Understanding the influence of age-related hormonal changes is essential for recognizing potential barriers to sexual function and pursuing strategies to maintain or enhance sexual health.

Holistic Approach to Hormonal Balance:

Maintaining healthy testosterone levels requires a holistic approach that encompasses various aspects of well-being.

Physical Activity: Regular exercise, particularly resistance and cardiovascular training, supports testosterone production. Engaging in physical activity enhances blood flow, stimulates hormone release, and contributes to overall vitality.

Nutrition: Consuming a balanced diet rich in essential nutrients, including zinc, vitamin D, and healthy fats, is fundamental for hormonal balance. These nutrients support hormone synthesis and overall well-being.

Stress Management: Chronic stress can disrupt hormonal balance and negatively impact testosterone levels. Engaging in stress-reduction techniques such as meditation, relaxation exercises, and mindfulness supports hormonal equilibrium.

As you gain insight into the intricate connection between testosterone and erectile function, you're empowered to make informed decisions about your sexual health journey. By embracing a holistic approach that encompasses lifestyle adjustments, open communication, and other strategies explored in this book, you're taking proactive steps to maintain optimal testosterone levels and enjoy a satisfying and fulfilling sexual life.

Natural Ways to Boost Testosterone Levels

Maintaining healthy testosterone levels is essential for optimal sexual health and overall vitality. This section delves into practical and effective methods to naturally boost testosterone levels, offering insights into lifestyle adjustments, dietary considerations, and stress management techniques that contribute to enhanced erectile function and well-being.

Healthy Lifestyle Choices:

Regular Exercise: Engaging in regular physical activity, especially strength training and cardiovascular exercises, supports testosterone production. Exercise stimulates hormone release, promotes blood circulation, and contributes to overall vitality.

Adequate Sleep: Prioritize quality sleep to support hormonal balance. Aim for 7-9 hours of uninterrupted sleep per night to optimize testosterone production and regulate hormonal rhythms.

Stress Management:

Mindfulness and Relaxation: Chronic stress elevates cortisol levels, which can impact testosterone production. Practicing mindfulness, deep breathing, meditation, and relaxation techniques reduces stress hormones and promotes hormonal equilibrium.

<u>Healthy Diet:</u>

Nutrient-Rich Foods: Consume a diet rich in nutrients that support testosterone production. Foods high in zinc, such as lean meats, nuts, and seeds, contribute to hormone synthesis. Vitamin D, found in fatty fish and fortified foods, also plays a crucial role in maintaining hormonal balance.

Omega-3 Fatty Acids: Incorporate foods rich in omega-3 fatty acids, like salmon and flaxseeds. Omega-3s support overall health and contribute to hormone regulation.

Antioxidant-Rich Foods: Consume antioxidant-rich foods, including fruits and vegetables, to combat oxidative stress and promote optimal hormonal function.

Dietary Considerations:

Limit Sugar and Processed Foods: High sugar intake and processed foods can lead to insulin resistance, negatively impacting hormone balance. Choose whole, unprocessed foods to support overall health and hormonal equilibrium.

Moderate Alcohol Consumption: Excessive alcohol consumption can suppress testosterone production. If you choose to consume alcohol, do so in moderation.

Balancing Hormones:

Body Composition: Achieving and maintaining a healthy body weight contributes to hormonal balance. Excess body fat, particularly abdominal fat, can lead to imbalances in hormone levels.

Hydration: Staying hydrated supports overall health and can help maintain hormonal balance.

<u>Consultation and Patience:</u>

Individual Responses: Remember that responses to lifestyle changes vary. Be patient and allow time for your body to adjust to new habits.

Consultation with Professionals: Before making significant changes to your lifestyle or diet, consult with healthcare professionals. They can offer personalized guidance based on your individual health status and needs.

By embracing these natural methods to boost testosterone levels, you're taking proactive steps toward enhancing your sexual health and overall well-being. These strategies, when integrated into a comprehensive approach that encompasses other aspects of sexual vitality, contribute to improved erectile function, increased libido, and a more satisfying and fulfilling sexual life.

When to Consider Hormone Therapy

Hormone therapy can be a valuable tool in addressing Erectile Dysfunction (ED) and hormonal imbalances that impact sexual health. However, considering hormone therapy requires careful assessment and understanding of when it may be an appropriate option. This section provides insights into the circumstances under which hormone therapy can be considered and guides readers toward making informed decisions.

Consultation with Healthcare Professionals:

Symptoms and Concerns: If you're experiencing persistent symptoms of ED, reduced libido, or other signs of hormonal imbalance, it's essential to consult healthcare professionals who specialize in hormonal health. These experts can evaluate your condition and recommend appropriate treatment options.

Medical History: Your medical history plays a significant role in determining whether hormone therapy is suitable for you. Conditions such as diabetes, heart disease, and certain cancers can influence the decision to undergo hormone therapy.

Exploring Other Options:

Lifestyle Adjustments: Before considering hormone therapy, explore lifestyle adjustments and natural methods to support hormonal balance. Engaging in regular exercise, maintaining a healthy diet, managing stress, and improving sleep can positively impact hormonal health.

Open Communication: Maintain open communication with your partner about your sexual health concerns and treatment options. Partner support and understanding can play a pivotal role in your decision-making process.

When to Consider Hormone Therapy:

Age-Related Hormonal Decline: Hormone therapy, such as Testosterone Replacement Therapy (TRT), may be considered when age-related declines in testosterone levels lead to significant symptoms, impacting libido, erectile function, and overall quality of life.

Medical Conditions: Individuals with medical conditions that contribute to hormonal imbalances, such as hypogonadism or other endocrine disorders, may benefit from hormone therapy under the guidance of healthcare professionals.

Lack of Response to Other Treatments: If lifestyle adjustments and other treatments have not effectively addressed hormonal imbalances or ED, hormone therapy could be a viable option to explore.

Consultation and Monitoring:

Medical Supervision: If you're considering hormone therapy, it's crucial to undergo treatment under the supervision of experienced healthcare professionals. They will assess your hormonal levels, monitor your progress, and adjust treatment plans as necessary.

Benefits and Risks: Understand the potential benefits and risks associated with hormone therapy. While hormone therapy can lead to improved libido, erectile function, and overall well-being, it's important to be aware of potential side effects and long-term implications.

Personal Decision: Deciding whether to pursue hormone therapy is a personal choice that requires careful consideration. Reflect on your individual health status, preferences, and goals when making this decision.

By gaining a clear understanding of when to consider hormone therapy, you're equipped to approach your sexual health journey with informed decision-making and a comprehensive approach. Remember that the ultimate goal is to achieve optimal sexual well-being and enjoy a satisfying and fulfilling sexual life. Consultation with healthcare professionals, thorough research, and open communication are essential components of this process.

Chapter 9: Creating Your Personalized Plan

we embark on the journey of crafting a personalized plan to address Erectile Dysfunction (ED) and promote optimal sexual health. This chapter guides you through the process of assessing your current lifestyle, building a holistic plan that caters to your unique needs, and implementing strategies to track your progress and make necessary adjustments.

Assessing Your Current Lifestyle and Habits

Before devising a personalized plan, it's essential to gain a comprehensive understanding of your current lifestyle and habits. This section encourages introspection and self-awareness, allowing you to identify factors that contribute to your sexual health and well-being.

Self-Reflection: Reflect on your daily routines, dietary choices, physical activity, stress levels, and sleep patterns. Identify any habits that might be influencing your sexual function.

Communication: Engage in open communication with your partner about your sexual health journey. Discuss any concerns, goals, and preferences that should be incorporated into your personalized plan.

Medical Evaluation: Seek medical evaluation from healthcare professionals who specialize in sexual health. This evaluation can provide insights into underlying factors contributing to ED and guide the development of your personalized plan.

Building a Holistic Plan Tailored to Your Needs

Once you have a clear understanding of your current situation, it's time to build a holistic plan that aligns with your unique needs and goals. This section helps you create a roadmap for enhancing your sexual health and well-being.

Setting Goals: Define clear and realistic goals for your sexual health journey. Whether it's improving erectile function, increasing libido, or enhancing overall intimacy, articulate your objectives.

Lifestyle Adjustments: Incorporate insights from previous chapters into your plan. Consider strategies such as communication techniques, stress reduction methods, dietary adjustments, and exercise routines.

Integration: Integrate various components of your personalized plan into your daily life. Create a structured approach that accounts for physical, emotional, and mental well-being.

Tracking Progress and Making Adjustments

Progress tracking and adjustment are crucial aspects of any effective plan. This section emphasizes the importance of monitoring your progress, celebrating successes, and making necessary adjustments to optimize your outcomes.

Documentation: Keep a journal or digital record of your journey. Document changes in sexual function, mood, energy levels, and overall well-being.

Regular Check-Ins: Schedule regular check-ins with healthcare professionals to assess your progress and address any concerns. Professional guidance ensures that your plan remains aligned with your evolving needs.

Flexibility: Be open to making adjustments based on your experiences. Your plan is not static; it should evolve as you gain insights and experience improvements.

Celebrating Successes: Acknowledge and celebrate the positive changes you experience along the way. Recognize that even small steps toward improvement are significant accomplishments.

Creating your personalized plan is an empowering step toward revitalizing your sexual health and overall well-being. By assessing your current lifestyle, building a holistic approach that aligns with your needs, and tracking your progress with a commitment to adjustments, you're embracing a journey of self-discovery and enhancement. Remember that every individual's path is unique; your personalized plan is a reflection of your preferences, aspirations, and determination to achieve optimal sexual vitality and satisfaction.

Conclusion

As you reach the conclusion of "Revive Your Manhood Naturally: A Guide to Fixing Erectile Dysfunction Naturally and Safely," it's evident that your journey toward enhanced sexual health and well-being has been enlightening and empowering. Throughout this comprehensive guide, you've explored the intricate aspects of Erectile Dysfunction (ED), delving into its causes, prevalence, and the wide range of holistic solutions available to you.

From understanding the role of hormones, exploring natural remedies, embracing mindfulness techniques, to considering hormone therapy when appropriate, you've gained valuable insights and practical strategies to revitalize your sexual vitality naturally. By adopting a holistic approach that encompasses lifestyle adjustments, open communication, and self-care, you're taking proactive steps toward achieving optimal erectile function and overall satisfaction in your sexual life.

Remember that your journey is unique, and progress takes time. Celebrate the small victories, acknowledge the positive changes you've experienced, and remain patient with yourself as you continue to implement the techniques and insights presented in this guide. Stay engaged in open communication with your partner and seek guidance from healthcare professionals as needed.

As you move forward, let your newfound knowledge and empowered mindset guide you toward a more fulfilling, vibrant, and satisfying sexual life. The journey doesn't end here—your commitment to your well-being will continue to lead you toward a brighter future filled with enhanced intimacy, connection, and confidence.

Thank you for embarking on this journey with "Revive Your Manhood Naturally." May your path to optimal sexual health be one of growth, transformation, and endless possibility.

Appendix

Additional Resources and References

In this appendix, you'll find a compilation of additional resources and references that can further enhance your understanding of Erectile Dysfunction (ED) and strategies for promoting sexual health. These resources provide in-depth information, expert insights, and avenues for continued learning.

Websites and Organizations:

American Urological Association (AUA): www.auanet.org

International Society for Sexual Medicine (ISSM): www.issm.info

National Institute of Diabetes and Digestive and Kidney Diseases (NIDDK): www.niddk.nih.gov

Mayo Clinic: www.mayoclinic.org

Glossary of Terms

Erectile Dysfunction (ED): The inability to achieve or sustain an erection sufficient for sexual activity.

Libido: Sexual desire or drive.

Testosterone: The primary male sex hormone responsible for various bodily functions, including sexual health.

Nitric Oxide: A molecule that relaxes blood vessel walls and promotes blood flow, crucial for achieving and maintaining erections.

Hormone Therapy: Medical treatment involving the administration of hormones to address imbalances or deficiencies.

Testosterone Replacement Therapy (TRT): A form of hormone therapy involving the supplementation of testosterone to alleviate symptoms of low testosterone levels.

Pelvic Floor Muscles: Muscles that support the pelvic organs, play a role in erectile function, and influence ejaculation.

Mindfulness: A practice that involves being fully present and engaged in the present moment.

Stress Management Techniques: Strategies such as deep breathing, meditation, and progressive muscle relaxation used to reduce stress and anxiety.

Holistic Approach: A comprehensive approach that addresses multiple aspects of well-being, including physical, emotional, and mental health.

Medical Supervision: Oversight by healthcare professionals to ensure safe and effective treatment.

Oxidative Stress: Imbalance between the production of harmful free radicals and the body's ability to counteract their effects.

Andropause: The gradual decline in testosterone levels that occurs as men age.

Consultation: Seeking guidance and advice from qualified healthcare professionals.

Acknowledging these terms: Understanding the terminology related to sexual health is essential for informed decision-making and effective communication with healthcare professionals. The glossary serves as a quick reference to key terms encountered throughout the book, ensuring clarity and comprehensive comprehension.

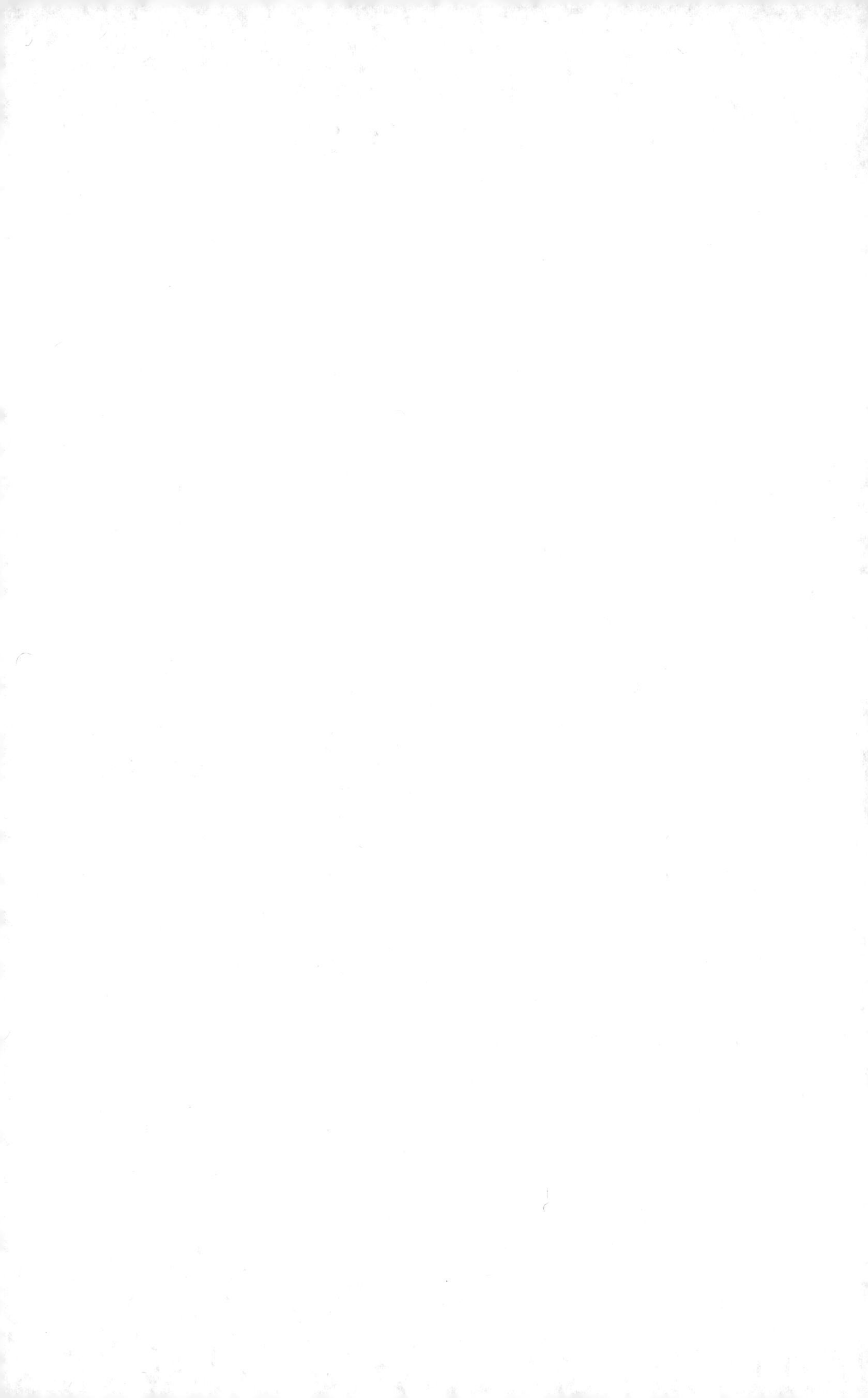

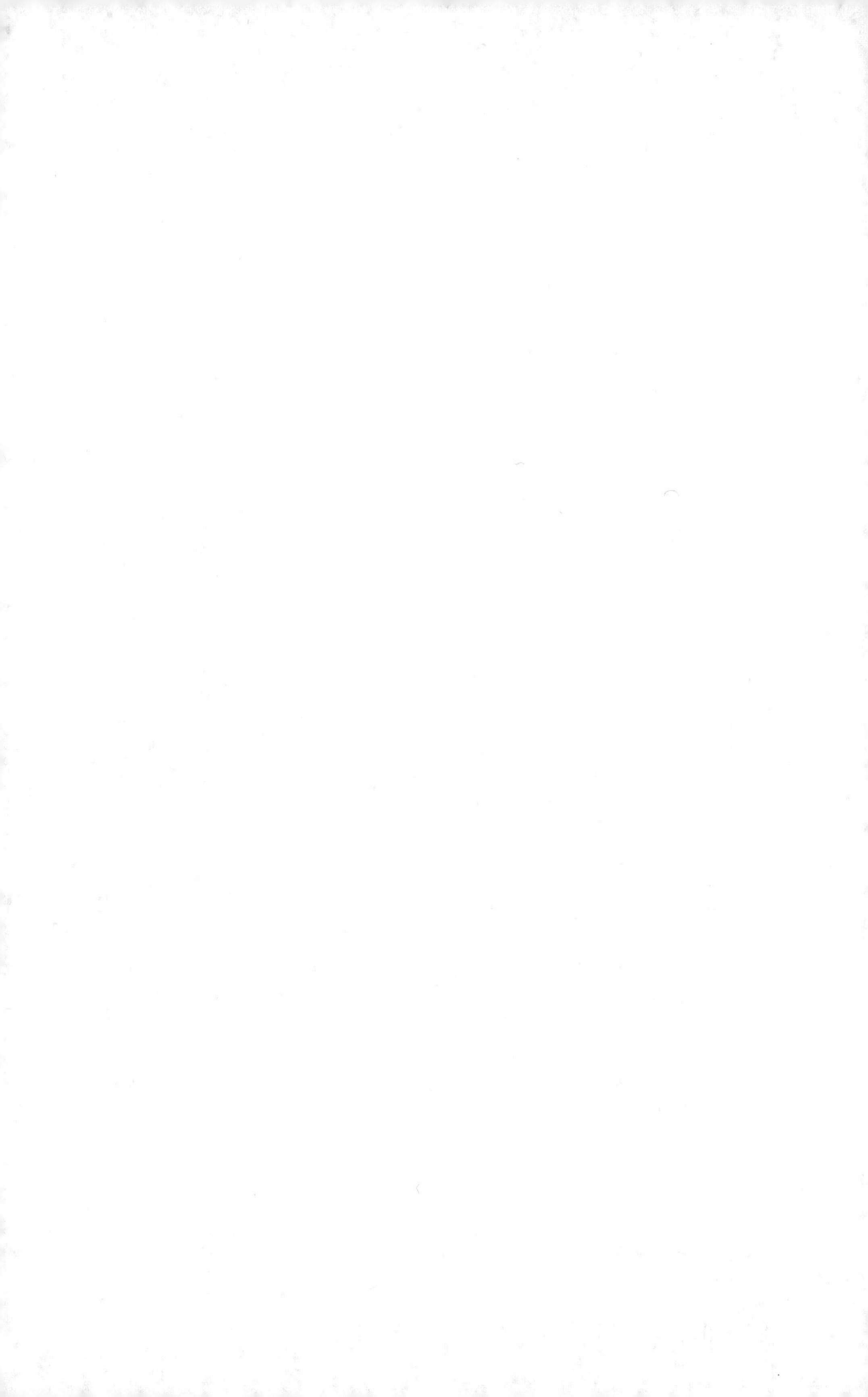